THE CAUSE OF AUTISM

VACCINES, ACETAMINOPHEN, INFLAMMATION

BY

DR. STEPHEN SCHULTZ, DDS, MS, MPH, PHD

The opinions expressed in this book are my own and do not necessarily coincide with those of any of the other individuals mentioned in this book.

TABLE OF CONTENTS

INTRODUCTION

In this sad world of ours sorrow comes to all, and to the young it comes with bittered agony because it takes them unawares. The older have learned to expect it. ~Abraham Lincoln

While getting my PhD in public health epidemiology at the University of California San Diego (UCSD) and San Diego State University (SDSU), I was often told by my professors: Do not ever say you have found the cause of a disease. Doing so is unprofessional and unrealistic. It takes many years of studies by many scientists to come to the conclusion that a cause for any particular disease has been found using the tools of epidemiology. Well, now after much research published on the subject, I am saying that I have found the cause for autism. Perhaps, that makes me a fool, or perhaps there is now enough evidence to make that statement. I will take the license and hope that I am not a fool.

For sixteen years now I have been saying that giving a child acetaminophen during early brain development is associated with autism. I even wrote my dissertation on this topic which was accepted by UCSD and SDSU in 2006. In 2008, I published an article based on this research in the prestigious journal *Autism: the International Journal of Research and Practice.* Although I initially was alone against the medical establishment in my belief in the effects of acetaminophen use causing autism (and feeling like David slinging stones at Goliath or perhaps more recently Dr. Strange vs. Thanos with me as Dr. Strange—some of my colleagues would say an apt moniker), I have been joined over the years by others, including more eminent scholars than myself. These days, I feel more like the blind Samson with his hands resting on the pillars, ready to bring the whole temple down. I believe there is sufficient evidence now to prove the acetaminophen/autism connection and will trust in the Almighty, as Samson did, and the future to bear me out.

I wanted to get the purpose of the book right up front here in the introduction. Those of you who just wanted to find that out can stop reading now. However, those of you who are intrigued and would like to hear more details, please continue reading. I like to think that there may be something else in this little book that you can grab onto as something useful for your life. As you will see, I also implicate vaccines and other forms of inflammation—as well as methods of autism prevention.

Of course, the title of this book really says it all. Autism is caused by the inflammation in the brain during development primarily from acetaminophen use and vaccines. In my humble way, I am presenting a way forward. I believe there is much we can do to prevent and treat autism.

I begin every section with a quotation from Abraham Lincoln, not only because I think he is the greatest president that America has produced (and paradoxically for today's politics the first Republican president), but also because his words live on as his legacy for us. He may be the most moral and humble statesman that America has ever produced, again a tremendous contrast for today. His words are as strikingly germane for us today as when he wrote them a century and a half ago during our nation's greatest trial. I am hopeful that they will be as inspirational to you as they continue to be for me.

I am of the opinion that the trying times that produced the Civil War 150 years ago are quite relevant to the situation we find ourselves in today. Not only did it produce Abraham Lincoln but also Ulysses S. Grant. His real name was Hiram Ulysses Grant, but he was too shy to correct the registrar when he was admitted to West Point. Picture if you will a shy young boy of seventeen with sweaty palms who, as he later wrote, did not think he possessed the requirements to study at West Point. There are many stories about how he was registered as U.S. Grant at West Point, but I think I may have hit on the real story. When asked his name by the registrar, he would have quietly said "Hiram Ulysses Grant" which the registrar would have heard as "I am Ulysses S. Grant."

He was an undistinguished student at West Point, except in mathematics where he discovered a real talent. On the parade field, he had trouble keeping step with the other soldiers to the martial music. He said of himself that he could recognize only two tunes, "One was Yankee Doodle," he said, "and the other wasn't." I find it interesting that he had difficulty understanding music. The mumps virus can infect the brain and cause hearing problems and even deafness. Could U.S. Grant's hearing problems have been caused by a mumps virus infection? It is curious that a mutated form of the mumps virus is included in the MMR vaccination.

Ever since he was young he loved working with horses, and his quiet manner could calm even the most disagreeable horse. Later when he was General Grant, he had a teamster tied to a tree for six hours for mistreating a horse. I believe it's safe to say that he loved horses more than most people, with the notable exceptions of his wife Julia, their four children, and his good friend General Sherman. General Sherman said of him that he had a simple faith in success and never worried about what the enemy was planning, while his own plans carried him through victory after victory. He had a tremenous ability to concentrate. Even in the midst of pandemonium in battle, he remained clear-headed and in charge. Because of his many victories in the west, General Grant was called to Washington by President Lincoln and promoted to the rank of Lieutenant General, the first to have that rank since George Washington. As he later wrote in his memoirs, he was very shy when the president invited him to a party at the White House. Everyone there wanted to get a look at him, and Edwin Stanton, the Secretary of War, stood him up on a sofa so that everyone could see him. He was very embarrassed and greatly afraid that they were going to ask him to give a speech. It was said of him that he could be silent in several languages.

I think it is possible that General Grant was "on the spectrum" of autism, and yet he rose above his limitations to win the Civil War and serve two terms as a very popular president who led us through the recostruction of our country. In fact, he was asked to run for a third term by the Republicans, but he politely declined. He wanted to travel to Europe with his beloved wife Julia. Although, he could have won again—he was that popular and admired. His reputation has been smeared for many years by southern historians who did not want to see black people treated fairly as equal citizens. They say his policies stopped the reconstruction of the southern way of life—which indeed it did—and that was a good thing. Now President Grant's reputation is undergoing a revival as more people have come to appreciate his reconstruction of the South which continued Abraham Lincoln's desire for freedom and equality for all Americans.

It's also interesting that President Grant also tried to secure the rights of Native Americans at a time when almost no one else cared about them. He invited their leaders to Washington to try to bring peace and honor the government's treaties—which had often been ignored by the US almost as soon as the ink had dried. I recently heard an interesting and sad theory about the decline in population of Native Americans. It is thought that so many of them died through disease brought by European immigrants and wars with the US government that it actually brought on climate change. The theory surmises that the decrease in wood-burning campfires decreased carbon dioxide in the atmosphere to bring on the Little Ice Age in Europe. Paradoxically, the crop failures that resulted caused even more immigrants to leave Europe for America.

Although I cannot say that I'm anywhere near as accomplished as President Grant was, I also possess some of his personality and am also quite possibly "on the spectrum." I too was drawn to mathematics, and much of the work I do as an epidemiologist is data analysis. I am loathe to admit this propensity even to myself because it also means that I have passed on some of these genes to my son with autism. As I see autism after many years of research, I believe it begins with a genetic predisposition which is then amplified by environmental factors such as infections, certain vaccinations (which are currently unknown and need to be investigated), and acetaminophen use which potentiates the inflammation and damages the endocannabinoid system. I will explore these in greater detail in the folowing chapters.

Abraham Lincoln said during the war that he was looking for a general who could understand the arithamatic. By this, he meant that his generals so far had not been able to accept the heavy losses required in the Civil War battles. He found his mathetician, but perhaps more litterally than he had intended, in General Grant who was able to look past the number of dead on the battlefield and keep right on fighting until victory.

I chose the Lincoln quote for the Introduction because it reminded me that autism begins at an early age and before children have experience to know that life is a struggle between sorrow and joy.

Chapter 1. My Mission

The Beginning

I have been driven many times upon my knees by the overwhelming conviction that I had nowhere else to go. My own wisdom and that of all about me seemed insufficient for that day. Adhere to your purpose and you will soon feel as well as you ever did. On the contrary, if you falter, and give up, you will lose the power of keeping any resolution, and will regret it all your life.   ~Abraham Lincoln

My son Nathan was a bright little boy and was already using ten words by the time of his first birthday. Every evening at this time he came over and sat with me in my easy chair while we both watched his favorite movies: sing-a-long movies from Disney. In his thirteenth month, Nathan had his first measles-mumps-rubella (MMR) vaccination. He became very ill with constant diarrhea and bloating. Then he broke out on his chest and stomach in a measles rash that lasted for several weeks. His doctor told us to give him acetaminophen and it seemed to ease his suffering. Gradually, he appeared to get better, but over the course of the following year, Nathan lost all speech, his sociability, and he preferred to sit alone on the floor. If I picked him up to watch a movie with me, he squirmed and fought until he got back on the floor. He wouldn't look at the TV or even appear to hear the songs. He was diagnosed with autism shortly after he reached the age of two. Actually, that's not quite correct. His pediatrician told me that he was on a spectrum and had "developmental delay not otherwise specified." I had no idea what that meant, but I imagine now that it was a way to let me down easy. The internet is a wonderful thing—I was able to figure out what he really meant—autism. Nathan's doctor could not tell me why Nathan had autism, so I began reading about autism and found that the cause was unknown.

There were many theories out there about the cause of autism: vaccinations, mercury in vaccinations, prescription medicines, mother's illness during pregnancy, childhood illness, environmental pollution, and many more. I thought that it might be the MMR vaccination or mercury in vaccines (although it's not in the MMR) since Nathan had shown his regression into autism after his MMR vaccination and, of course, he had many other vaccinations he had around the same time. I wanted to to find out what happened to my son and also if that knowledge might render a treatment. I realized, too, that there were many other children similarly afflicted and in ever increasing numbers. I wanted to help stop this epidemic and, God willing, find a treatment, since there was none that seemed to work well, and though I scarcely wished to hope for it, a cure.

Like Lincoln, I found myself on my knees praying to God to let me help my son and others like him. Abraham Lincoln's quote at the beginning of this chapter seemed appropriate. I will take his advice and not falter, so that I will not regret it all my life.

MY QUEST

I know not how to aid you, save in the assurance of one of mature age, and much severe experience, that you cannot fail, if you resolutely determine, that you will not. ~Abraham Lincoln

Since the cause of autism was unknown and there was no effective treatment, I decided that it was my personal responsibility to go back to school to discover the cause of my son's autism and see if I could find a way to help him. At the time, I was in the Navy and performing research at the Naval Dental Research Institute (NDRI) at Great Lakes Naval Base just north of Chicago, Illinois. I applied to the Navy to select me for Duty Under Instruction for two years to study for a masters of public health degree followed by a one year residency at the National Institutes of Health. I was selected to begin my quest at the Uniformed Services

University of the Health Sciences (USUHS). After that, I never looked back.

As in the Lincoln quote above that I chose for this section, I resolutely determined not to fail, and trusted in God and the wisdom of Abraham Lincoln that I would not— although I was also getting close to the mature age of our beloved president, and also feeling the pangs of my own severe experience, as any parent of a child with autism can attest. President Lincoln was 56 when he died (although the war had aged him beyond his years), and I am now 64, soon to be 65, and believe that I can finally say that I have not failed my son. I know how my son came to have autism, and I know the path that can lead to an effective biomedical treatment.

MY QUALIFICATIONS

I hold that while man exists, it is his duty to improve not only his own condition, but to assist in ameliorating mankind. ~Abraham Lincoln

I was not totally unprepared for the challenge that presented itself to me. When I began, I had a Bachelor of Science (BS) degree in microbiology and a Master of Science (MS) in biology from the University of Illinois— Urbana, Illinois, and I stayed an extra year there studying genetics. This was followed by a Doctor of Dental Surgery

(DDS) degree and an extra bachelor's degree, this time in dentistry, from the University of Illinois at the Medical Center (UIMC), now joined to the University of Illinois—Chicago. Additionally, I was presented an award at graduation from the American Academy of Oral Pathology while receiving my DDS degree for research I performed in the oral pathology department at the UIMC School of Dentistry. Those were all of my initial qualifications when my son first showed signs of autism. It wasn't perhaps enough to make a real dent in autism research, but I thought perhaps with a little more education, I could make a more qualified effort.

I continued my education seventeen years later when my son with autism was three years old, not knowing if I still had enough brain power to learn and graduate again. But I was still able to study (Thank God) and receive a Master of Public Health (MPH) degree with a specialization in epidemiology after one year of preparation at the Uniformed Services University of the Health Sciences, mercifully known as USUHS pronounced you-sus. Some of the more unkind members of the military would like to pronounce it use-less, but I beg their pardon and refuse the license.

This was followed by a residency and fellowship in public health (I was given certificates for both) at the National Institutes of Health (NIH), specifically the National Institute of Dental and Craniofacial Research (NIDCR). This was followed by a two year hiatus from school where I actually had to do some work at the Naval Dental Center Southwest in San Diego. By the way, San Diego, in my humble opinion has the best weather in the US. When I applied and was selected by the Navy to again go back to school, I elected to stay in San Diego. This time the Navy paid for me to attend school for four years. (Some of the more astute of my Navy friends said they were going to keep sending me back to school until I finally learned to do something useful.) This time I earned a Doctor of Philosophy (PhD) degree in public health epidemiology by studying at San Diego State University (SDSU) for the first year and the University of California San Diego (UCSD) for the final three years in a joint doctoral program between the two universities. There were 25 years between my DDS and PhD degrees (1981-2006), but I guess old age had not stopped my brain from working. I finally learned enough—the Navy stopped sending me back to school— and I felt I finally knew enough to make an informed effort to study and publish scientific articles on autism, while still fulfilling my duties wherever the Navy sent me.

I chose the Lincoln quote for this chapter because this is what I have tried to do. I have tried to improve my condition with education, so that I can assist in helping my son and others with autism.

Chapter 2.   It's Not Mercury

I never encourage deceit, and falsehood, especially if you have got a bad memory, is the worst enemy a fellow can have. The fact is truth is your truest friend, no matter what the circumstances are.   ~Abraham Lincoln

While attending USUHS, I spent many hours in their library reading journal articles about autism with the enthusiasm of a student currently being schooled in epidemiology and SAS statistical programming. This was augmented by the fact that I now had access to full journal articles, as the library was well-appointed with journal access both in bound form and on their computers. My first inclination was that mercury in vaccinations was the cause of my son's autism. I had been working at NDRI on a project to remove mercury contamination from the environment. I knew that it's a poison and could cause brain damage. Could the small amounts of mercury preservative added to some vaccines cause the brain damage we call autism?

I was able to thoroughly examine the issue of whether mercury in vaccinations was the cause for my son's autism. After judicious and rigorous reading, I determined that it was not mercury. The most potent argument in my own mind which exonerated mercury from this role was that even after the preservative was removed from vaccines, the incidence of autism continued to increase.

Some people clung to the idea that trace amounts of mercury still in vaccines could cause autism. Others insisted that environmental mercury from coal-burning power plants or from dental treatment was autism's cause, but I moved on. It was time to investigate other possibilities.

Having had much experience researching this topic, I was requested some years later to author a review article on this subject by the editor of the prestigious journal *Acta Neurobiologica Eperimentalis* of the Nencki Institute of Experimental Biology and the Polish Neuroscience Society. I wrote for them an article which I entitled "Does thimerosal or other mercury exposure increase the risk for autism? A review of current literature." This article was published by this journal in 2010, and is available for free through the US National Library of Medicine:

https://www.ncbi.nlm.nih.gov/pubmed/20628442

I thought the quote from Abraham Lincoln for this chapter to be most appropriate due to the feelings of bitterness I felt from some of my colleagues when my paper was published. I believed that I had fairly weighed the balance of the published literature and found that the bulk of it exonerated mercury in the cause of autism. I am reminded of the writing on the wall which was interpreted by Daniel in the Bible to mean: "You are weighed in the balance and found wanting." Evidence for mercury was "found wanting" for causing autism. Some of my colleagues were deeply disturbed by this finding and still clung to what I had shown to be erroneous beliefs.

I chose the Lincoln quote for this chapter because I found many researchers unable to change their opinions regarding mercury/autism connection. When the evidence showed no connection, some researchers refused to give up—perhaps because they'd spent so long arguing that there was a connection. I believe when the evidence is against a theory, it's time to re-evaluate and move on.

CHAPTER 3. MEASLES-MUMPS-RUBELLA VACCINATION

I am a firm believer in the people. If given the truth, they can be depended upon to meet any national crisis. The great point is to bring them the real facts. ~Abraham Lincoln

I knew that my son's autism began after the measles-mumps-rubella (MMR) vaccination. I had already explored and rejected mercury as a cause for his condition, and I knew there was no mercury in this vaccination. Could it be that the MMR vaccination itself was the problem? By this time, I had finished my MPH degree at USUHS and had begun a residency/postdoc at the National Institutes of Health (NIH) to study public health, further my education in SAS statistical programming, and practice my recently learned epidemiology skills at the National Institute of Dental and Craniofacial Research (NIDCR).

The MMR vaccination contains live attenuated strains of measles virus, mumps virus, and rubella virus. I researched all three of these viruses at NIDCR, gradually focusing in on the mumps virus. I know what most people would say: "The mumps virus is harmless. It causes a mild infection of the salivary glands, especially the parotid, and is self-limiting. It may also get into the cerebral spinal fluid, but rarely does it cause any lasting problems."

That is true of the wild-type virus—children usually only get mildly ill and then get better. But what does that mean in terms of evolution? It means the mumps virus has been with us for many many years—so long that it knows not to produce severe illness that will kill its host and prevent its spread to naïve individuals in the population. But science has "improved" this virus through mutations, so that it no longer produces this short acute illness. It does, however, produce chronic illness—long-lasting infected for a lifetime kind of chronic illness. It's a sad truth that all three of the viruses in the MMR produce a long-lasting and frequently lifetime chronic infections. This is the dirty little secret about live viral vaccines: They are designed to give children a chronic infection forever—which is how they can give lifetime immunity. And sadly, the new and improved mumps virus also infects the brain—maybe also forever. Are we playing God with these viruses—mutating them to our will without knowing the long-term side effects?

I presented the results of my research on the MMR vaccination as my required residency/postdoc research presentation at NIDCR. I had been able to establish, albeit tenuously, an association of the MMR vaccination to autism using data from the National Health Interview Survey from NIH.

But you may be thinking: "The MMR vaccine has been tested for safety. We don't need to worry about it. All those parents who claim their child developed autism after the MMR are delusional. It only seems like there is a problem with the MMR vaccine because autism is usually diagnosed around the same time that the MMR is given." Unfortunately for this point of view is that there are no long-term safety tests on any vaccines given to children. To say that another way, children given a new vaccine are only tested short-term to see if there are any immediate problems (and make sure there is a great antibody response).

The Food and Drug Administration (FDA) does not require any long-term testing before approving a new vaccine. No one would ever discover if a child develops autism (or any other disease) a year after vaccination. The FDA is interested in short-term problems that develop in a clinical trial as well as how well the vaccine prevents the illness it has been designed to prevent.

The MMR is great at preventing acute measles, mumps, and rubella infections, since vaccinated individuals are already chronically infected! This may come as a shock to you as it did to me, but I assure you that this is true. While getting my PhD, I verified this fact with my immunology professor. This chronic infection cannot be good for the developing brains of infants.

In Japan, they no longer use the MMR vaccine. It was discontinued from use in 1993 because mumps virus component caused aseptic meningitis. This is a brain infection caused by just one of the live viruses in the MMR. Interestingly, this complication was more frequent in males than in females—as is also found in autism. Does the genetically modified mumps virus found in the MMR used in the US also cause aseptic meningitis, and does this infection lead to autism? We don't know because the study has not been done. What we do know is scary, because mumps virus has a predilection for brain infection which would lead to brain inflammation. Maybe they are smarter than we are in Japan—they have not gone back to the MMR vaccination and it has been now 26 years later.

I read with interest the article in the Journal of Pediatrics by DeStefano and colleagues in the Immunization Safety Office at the Centers for Disease Control and Prevention (CDC). It purports to exonerate the MMR vaccination and all other vaccines from any autism risk. It does not!

First of all, the study is overmatched, as reported by Dr. DeSoto at the University of Northern Iowa in her rebuttal to this article which is also in the same issue of the Journal of Pediatrics. In other words, when you match the cases and controls in a study on variables that affect exposure, then you will not see the true difference in exposure. In this case, the children were matched on variables that affect the amount of exposure to antibody-stimulating proteins and polysaccharides. It is not surprising that they saw no difference in the amount of these substances. Was it planned that way? It certainly makes one wonder if they had the results already in mind before they conducted the study.

The second reason it does not is in the title: Increasing Exposure to Antibody-Stimulating Proteins and Polysaccharides in Vaccines is Not Associated with Risk for Autism. Where in here does it say anything about the genetically altered measles, mumps, and rubella viruses in the MMR? It does not seem to cover that. Do the authors understand that these are live viruses being injected into our children? Do they understand that these genetically modified viruses have been selected to produce immediate and continuing lifelong inflammation? It does not matter that there are only 24 antigens per dose of MMR vaccine. These are live measles, mumps, and rubella viruses, and they will reproduce exponentially to produce millions of new viruses. Anyone with a little knowledge of microbiology or immunology would know that. Are the authors being intentionally misleading—aka lying? Or perhaps they are just proposing an "alternate truth." Did they measure the antibody response in the children they were studying? The thing that is truly important is the amount of brain inflammation caused by these vaccines, given alone or in combination, because brain inflammation is what is important for the development of autism. Did they measure the amount of interleukin 6 (IL-6) or other cytokines in the cerebral spinal fluid to determine the amount of brain inflammation caused by these vaccines? They did not!

The next reason this study is worthless is because it does not include the amount of adjuvants added to the vaccines to increase their inflammatory potential. The amount and type of these adjuvants is critical to the vaccine's ability to produce the greatest inflammatory and, therefore, antibody reaction. This information is readily available from the manufactures of vaccines. Do the authors account for the adjuvants used? Incredibly, they did not!

The important thing that is not even addressed in this study: What was the reaction of the cases and controls in this study to the vaccines they received? Were the children given acetaminophen if they had a bad reaction such as fever, measles rash, diarrhea, or irritability? The CDC itself lists these as common side effects of the MMR vaccination. The combination of a side effect and treatment with acetaminophen greatly increases the risk for autism, as I have shown in my PhD dissertation and 2008 paper. I will expand on this subject in the following chapter.

The final reason may seem elitist, but it is not intended to be. It is a matter of fact that none of these authors have a PhD degree in epidemiology or in any other subject. None of these authors has a research degree higher than the masters level. They should have had someone with a doctoral degree in epidemiology or statistics as an author (or at the very least a consultant) on their study. These authors made many errors and were not qualified to claim that there is no association between vaccination with the MMR or any other vaccine and the risk for autism. Is this study really the best we can expect from the Immunization Safety Office of the Centers for Disease Control and Prevention? Did the authors undertake this study with an open mind or did they already have a preconceived notion that all vaccines are good and the more vaccines the better!

Oh, and about that public health emergency in Washington state... On January 25, 2019, the governor declared a state-wide emergency due to a measles outbreak. At the time, there were 25 cases of measles, a number which has grown to 66 as of February 25th. I do not want to downplay the suffering of children (or adults, although most are children) who have contracted measles, but does that number of cases represent an emergency? You might ask as I did, how many children have died in this emergency? The answer is none. In fact, **there have been no deaths from measles in this country since 2015**. Yet, emergency vaccination centers have been set up to make sure everyone gets the MMR. And sadly, public health officials are now saying a child needs only to be six months old (rather than the usual 12 months old) to get the vaccine. This emergency is similar to the "emergency" at our southern US border. It is designed to push a political agenda rather than actually helping people.

I am not against vaccination, but we must balance that risk against the risk of causing harm in children while their brains are in a critical period of development. Studies must be done to determine the appropriate age to vaccinate and still reduce the risk of autism to a minimum. In other words, the risks must be balanced.

I chose the Lincoln quote for this chapter because I firmly believe that people will demand more research on the MMR vaccine when they are given the whole truth.

CHAPTER 4. IT'S NOT THE MMR VACCINE ALONE, BUT WORKING TOGETHER WITH ACETAMINOPHEN

Without the assistance of that Divine Being … I cannot succeed. With that assistance, I cannot fail.

~ Abraham Lincoln

After showing promise in research and completing my Masters Degree in Public Health with a one year residency/postdoc at NIH, I was sent to Naval Dental Center Southwest (NDCSW) in San Diego to do some actual work for the Navy for two years. I began those two years by being named Head, Public Health Department for NDCSW where I was rapidly promoted to the position of Director for Corporate Performance. I was in that position for only a short time, however. The Duty Under Instruction Board for the Navy selected me a second time to go back to school. The Admiral there was not happy to lose me, but realized the necessity of letting me go after I was selected by Naval headquarters in Washington DC to pursue a PhD degree.

The Navy allowed me to get a PhD of my choice—I chose to study public health epidemiology so that I could follow my quest to discover the cause of autism while still providing the public health support desired by the Navy. I began this research program with a great deal of trepidation—I was the oldest student in my class, having reached the age of 48. I wasn't sure I still had the brainpower to succeed, especially in the plethora of statistics classes I would need. Fortunately, I had friends there to help me.

My dissertation topic was "Environmental Risk Factors for Autistic Disorder." I presented my findings in a presentation to students and faculty in 2006. From this research, I was able to publish my paper in 2008 showing the increased risk for autism from a combination of the MMR vaccination and acetaminophen use. My paper was published in *Autism, the International Journal of Research and Practice*, the publication of the National Autistic Society in the UK. This paper is available through the US National Library of Medicine at:

https://www.ncbi.nlm.nih.gov/pubmed/18445737

Recently several studies have confirmed my earlier work that acetaminophen use increases the risk for autism. The most recent review of the subject of acetaminophen and autism risk is from the American Journal of Epidemiology in 2018: "Prenatal Exposure to Acetaminophen and Risk for Attention Deficit Hyperactivity Disorder and Autistic Spectrum Disorder: A Systematic Review, Meta-analysis, and Meta-regression Analysis of Cohort Studies" by Masarwa R, Levine H, Gorelik E, et al.

As Abraham Lincoln is quoted at the beginning of this chapter, with the assistance of the Divine Being, I too could not fail. I would add to that a quote from the Beatles; sometimes I needed to "get by with a little help from my friends."

Chapter 5. Coal Tar Analgesics: Acetanilide, Phenacetin, and Acetaminophen

If we could first know where we are, and whither we are tending, we could better judge what to do, and how to do it. ~Abraham Lincoln

In 2011, I was asked to give a presentation at the University of Texas Health Science Center in San Antonio regarding the use of acetaminophen and its association with autism. First I gave a brief summary of the history of acetaminophen use, and then gave my humble opinion of how acetaminophen may act to increase the risk for autism. A summary of the presentation follows and the full presentation is available on my blog at autismrisk.blog.

Two anti-fever agents were developed in the 1880s from coal tar: acetanilide in 1886 and phenacetin in 1887. In 1893, acetaminophen was discovered in the urine of individuals who had taken phenacetin, and was concentrated into a white, crystalline compound with a bitter taste. I'm not sure how they enticed people to try these compounds in the era before institutional review boards, but it seems amazing to me that anyone would willingly take a compound derived from coal tar without knowing what the results might be.

Eventually, acetanilide use was discontinued due to unacceptable toxic effects, the most alarming being cyanosis due to methemoglobinemia. Acetanilide turns blood a chocolate brown color as it methylates the hemoglobin in red blood cells. This reaction occurs in poisoning by acetanilide, phenacetin, nitrate, nitrate aniline dyes, and over 100 other compounds.

Although it was known that phenacetin could cause methemoglobinemia, the U.S. Food and Drug Administration did not order the withdrawal of drugs containing phenacetin until 1983, according to the Federal Register. By then, other side effects were being reported such as cancer and kidney damage.

Acetaminophen, which was found to be the active metabolite of acetanilide and phenacetin, was thought to be a safer alternative. Unfortunately, it causes three times as many cases of liver failure as all other drugs combined, and is the most common cause of acute liver failure in the United States, accounting for 39% of cases. While this kind of acetaminophen damage occurs through overdosing, even recommended doses, especially combined with even small amounts of alcohol, have caused irreversible liver failure.

Acetaminophen is a drug that relieves pain and fever and can be found in both prescription and over-the-counter (OTC) products. It is combined in many prescription products with other ingredients, usually opioids such as codeine (Tylenol with Codeine), oxycodone (Percocet), and hydrocodone (Vicodin).

The U.S. Food and Drug Administration (FDA) started restricting the use of acetaminophen starting in January of 2011. They asked manufacturers of prescription combination products that contain acetaminophen to limit the amount of acetaminophen to no more than 325 milligrams in each tablet or capsule. They also required manufacturers to update labels of all prescription combination acetaminophen products to warn of the potential risk for severe liver injury.

Acetaminophen is the last of the coal tar analgesics which is still available, and it too should be banned—at the very least banned for use in children. As I show in the next chapter, acetaminophen use is correlated with the beginning of the autism epidemic.

I chose the quote from Abraham Lincoln for this chapter because we need to know where we are in regards to acetaminophen use. My contention is that acetaminophen may be safe in small doses for some individuals in the short term but not for a child or developing fetus, especially when the immune system is being challenged by a vaccination such as the MMR.

As President Lincoln said, first we need to know where we are. In this case, we are prescribing a toxic chemical to children which I believe started the autism epidemic.

CHAPTER 6. ACETAMINOPHEN AND AUTISM

The true rule, in determining to embrace, or reject any thing, is not whether it have any evil in it; but whether it have more of evil, than of good. ~Abraham Lincoln

When I first considered whether acetaminophen use could increase the risk for autism, I remembered that my son got very sick from the MMR vaccination and was given acetaminophen prescribed in high doses by his pediatrician. I was wondering how I could test this theory—perhaps using a natural experiment.

Then I remembered that there were in 1982 and again in 1986 random poisonings by one or more individuals (the number of poisoners is not known because the cases were never solved) tampering with the contents of acetaminophen capsules. Capsules of acetaminophen had their contents removed and replaced with cyanide poison. This was easy to do at the time because packages were not so well sealed as they are today. In fact, these poisonings led to the more secure packaging that we have in place today. But in those more innocent times, capsules could be pulled apart and refilled easily, then placed back in their containers and placed on store shelves. Seven people were murdered this way in 1982. Acetaminophen capsules were recalled and sales of all acetaminophen products plummeted. Then things were allowed to get back to normal until 1986, when a woman was murdered in New York, again with cyanide-laced acetaminophen. Again sales of acetaminophen products plummeted. This time, the maker of acetaminophen sealed their capsules into "caplets" and produced more resistant packaging. The sales of acetaminophen products again resumed and continued to increase.

These two events, cruel and deadly though they were, were a natural experiment that I could exploit. I found a graph of the number of persons with Autistic Disorder enrolled by year of birth with the California Department of Developmental Services in their 1998 report to the legislature. When I saw the decreases which began in 1982 and 1986, I knew I was on to something. I found two other events which influenced acetaminophen sales in 1977 and 1980, both of which indicated acetaminophen sales correlated with autism cases.

The inflection point in 1980 is especially important. The number of persons with autism seems to be growing at a slow but steady pace—following population increases from 1961 until 1980. But in 1980, the US government decided that children should not be given aspirin due to the threat of Reye Syndrome, and warning labels were put on aspirin bottles to that effect. Parents were told that acetaminophen was the safe choice for use in children.

The change seen is immediate with the autism rate increasing significantly and substantially after that warning. Paradoxically, recent research indicates that there may never have been a Reye Syndrome threat after all.

The following figure graphically shows the changes in the numbers of autism cases dependent on these events.

Figure 1. Number of enrolled persons with autistic disorder in California by year of birth* with addition of events in the history of acetaminophen.

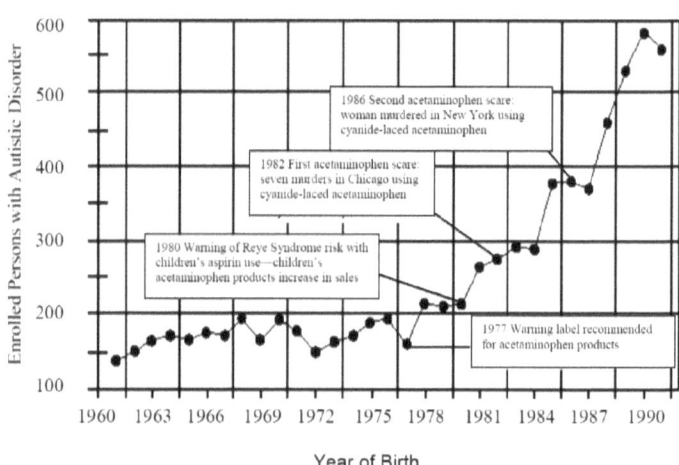

*From the California Department of Developmental Services

The graph reprinted here as Figure 1 is from a paper I published in 2010 with Dr. Kevin Becker of the Gene

Expression and Genomics Unit, National Institute on Aging, National Institutes of Health, and is available for free from the US National Library of Medicine at:

https://www.ncbi.nlm.nih.gov/pmc/articles/PMC3261751/

A recent paper, published on April 24, 2018 in the *American Journal of Epidemiology*, found a 20% increase in autism and a 30% increase in Attention Deficit Hyperactivity Disorder (ADHD) for mothers who took acetaminophen during pregnancy. This adds to the flood of recent papers exposing the dangers of acetaminophen use. I can almost hear the pillars cracking under the force of Samson's power.

Acetaminophen may—emphasis on *may*—be useful in some conditions in older adults, although it is very easy to take an overdose and risk liver damage. However, it is always a dangerous risk to expose children to it, even prenatally, while their brains are developing.

The Lincoln quote I chose for this chapter shows how I feel about acetaminophen. I believe it has more evil in it than good and its use should be rejected. At the very least, it should be made a prescription-only drug for adult use only.

CHAPTER 7. VACCINATIONS

You can fool all the people some of the time, and some of the people all the time, but you can not fool all the people all of the time. ~Abraham Lincoln

I have come to believe that it is a very peculiar idea to introduce live, albeit attenuated, viruses into young children. Some of you may remember that there was a time when this was not done. The first live attenuated virus that I was given as a child was the oral polio vaccine (OPV). I remember going down to my school with my family and getting a drop of vaccine on a sugar cube. It seemed like such a great idea until it began causing polio, including paralytic polio, in some vaccinees. It has since been replaced on the U.S. vaccination schedule by the inactivated polio vaccine (IPV). I would say that this is a wise precaution, although some stalwarts would say that the live oral vaccine causes better immunity, costs less, and is suitable for developing countries because it can be spread from vaccines to naïve individuals. I disagree. If it is not safe enough for Americans, how can it be safe enough for others?

More recently, the new live viral shingles vaccine has been coming under fire. It was supposed to be this great advancement to prevent reactivation of the chicken pox virus that causes shingles. But the National Vaccine Information Center reports, "Using the MedAlerts search engine, as of October 31, 2017, there have been more than 34,874 reports of shingles vaccine reactions, hospitalizations, injuries and deaths following shingles vaccinations made to the federal Vaccine Adverse Events Reporting System (VAERS), including 114 related deaths, 775 hospitalizations, and 562 related disabilities."

Perhaps some of these side effects are not really associated with the vaccine, but could it not be associated with some of them? A careful study should be conducted to see if the benefits from shingles vaccinations outweigh the risks. In fact, I believe I would not be wrong is saying that all vaccines should be tested in this way, especially if these vaccines are to be given to children.

Some of you may remember that early in 2017 our new president asked Robert F. (Bobby) Kennedy, Jr. to look into the safety of vaccinations. The rumor was that the president's son had a mild form of autism which might have been from a vaccination. Bobby Kennedy Jr. has been an outspoken advocate for this issue and is associated with the group SafeMinds which is very concerned about whether there is evidence that vaccinations are associated with the autism epidemic.

When I heard this, I volunteered to help any way I could. I had some experience in this area from a paper I had published in 2008, linking autism to acetaminophen use after the MMR vaccination. Also, I was very interested to delve more deeply into this possibility.

They asked me to review a group of eight articles that were presented to them as proof that vaccinations do not cause autism. Unfortunately, I did not find reassurance in the safety of vaccinations from these articles. In my humble opinion, none of them provided definitive evidence to exonerate vaccines from an association with autism risk. The following are the reviews that I provided for them.

These reviews and more of my research are available on my new blog autismrisk.blog and comments can be made on the blog or sent to autismriskresearch@gmail.com.

Review of Jain et al.: Autism Occurrence by MMR Vaccine Status Among US Children With Older Siblings With and Without Autism

This study seems to have been designed to show that younger siblings of children with autism (also called Augism Spectrum Disorder or ASD) are less likely to receive the MMR vaccine. As shown in their table 2, this is only seen at age 5 before the authors adjusted their model for covariates. The p value for this association is .003 before adjustment and .07 after adjustment. Since the p value is >.05 after adjustment, the authors have lost their significant finding. This is probably due to over-adjusting their model by including so many non-significant covariates.

However, they use this same dataset to try and determine if there is significant risk for ASD from MMR vaccination. There is a problem with doing this since there is a significant genetic component to autism risk as well as potentially similar environmental exposures between siblings. This would have an unknown effect on the association of MMR and ASD. The authors should have used their complete dataset to review the relationship of MMR to ASD in all children without limiting their review to risk among siblings.

A second problem with this study is the use of insurance data to establish their cases. ASD is better established by standardized testing. Using this dataset would lead to misclassification bias. In other words, the validity of identifying individuals with ASD is questionable.

A third, and I think crucial, problem with this study is the lack of information regarding other potential environmental risk factors. Many of these risk factors have been identified in the literature and could confound the association of MMR and ASD. The one that I find particularly important is the lack of information on acetaminophen use after vaccination which I have found to be important in my research.

Review of Yota et al.: Early exposure to the combined measles–mumps–rubella vaccine and thimerosal-containing vaccines and risk of autism spectrum disorder

The MMR vaccine used in Japan was different from the one used in the United States. Specifically, the mumps virus strain used in Japan was the Urabe strain the mumps virus and the strain used in the US was Jeryl Lynn (subsequently found to consist of two separate strains). For this reason, estimation of ASD risk from MMR use in the US vs. Japan will not give the same results. Additionally, the Japanese government stopped recommending MMR vaccine because its use was linked to aseptic meningitis thought to have been caused by the Urabe mumps strain. Imagine that! Their government stopped the use of the MMR because it caused an infection of the brain's meninges!

Further complicating the comparison of the US to Japan is the continuing use of monovalent measles, mumps, and rubella vaccines in Japan which was not accounted for in the study analysis in table 1. Parents could choose these monovalent vaccines instead of the MMR, and there is no accounting for when and how many of these vaccines were administered. Also, there is no mention of whether these vaccines contained thimerosal and should have been added to the mercury total in table 2 of the paper.

Additionally, the authors state that features of ASD are always present before the age of 3, which differs from the CDC website which states that ASD is usually diagnosed before the age of 6. If the authors only considered ASD diagnosed before the age of 3, this could lead to misclassification bias.

Finally, there is no mention of data collection for other environmental risk factors which could have confounded the association of MMR and ASD. Of particular concern from my research is the use of acetaminophen for any illness after MMR or monovalent vaccinations.

Review of Luke et al.: Vaccines are not associated with autism: An evidence-based meta-analysis of case-control and cohort studies

First it should be understood that this is a meta-analysis and not a study. In other words, it is a systematic review of published studies. The first problem I see with this paper is the small number of studies included in their meta analysis. Of the 1,112 studies identified and screened for retrieval, only 10 were actually used in the final analysis. This means that the authors rejected more than 99% of identified studies. Of the 10 studies the authors accepted, none showed an increased risk of ASD with MMR vaccination, mercury, or other vaccinations. It is not surprising that the meta-analysis of these 10 studies also found no increased risk of ASD from vaccinations. It is very easy to show no association when you can cherry pick your studies.

Another problem is that the authors decided only to include cohort and case-control studies. No randomized controlled trials were included. In addition, the authors reported that they decided not to include unpublished data. According to the published guide "How to Review a Meta-analysis" by Mark W. Russo, MD, MPH published in Gastroenterology and Hepatology, attempts should be made to collect unpublished data when performing a meta-analysis. Dr. Russo goes on to state "In high-quality meta-analyses, a standardized data abstraction form is developed and utilized by the authors and may be provided in the paper as a figure." No data abstraction form was provided in this meta-analysis.

Also, since this was a meta-analysis, there were no other environmental risk factors considered which may have confounded the association of vaccinations and ASD. A review of medications, including acetaminophen, taken by children during the period of vaccination could have yielded interesting results.

Review of Stoner et al. Patches of Disorganization in the Neocortex of Children with Autism

This is an excellent study that has been well planned and conducted. The results present a new understanding of the underlying brain organization prevalent in autism that may well point future research in the right direction of prevention and treatment. However, there are a few comments that need to be made regarding this study.

This study had a small sample size (11 cases and 11 controls) and this is a limitation of the study. Studying a larger number of cases and controls may show patches in more control children. Studying additional blocks from the sampled brains may also identify additional brain areas with patches. However, brain tissue samples from children are difficult to obtain, and the authors used samples from almost all of the subjects available to them from brain tissue banks.

The authors have described patches of disorganization in the neocortex in what they term "patch phenotype." These patches were observed predominantly in the brains of children with autism. However, one boy with autism had no observed patches and a patch was observed in a normally developing girl. In other words, having these patches may not be necessary nor sufficient to develop autism.

The authors do not conclude that autism necessarily begins prenatally but that prenatal processes do confer a predisposition to autism. In fact, all of the individuals whose brain tissue was examined were at least 2 years old when they died and there was no examination of prenatal brains. It should not be concluded that autism is a genetic disease based on identification of these patches. Indeed, it has been shown in a recent study that genetic factors and environment factors each contribute almost equally to the development of autism (Sandin et al., JAMA 2014). This study should not be used as proof that childhood vaccinations produce no risk for autism.

Review of Packer: Neocortical neurogenesis and the etiology of autism spectrum disorder

This is an interesting article reviewing neocortical neurogenesis in ASD through genetic variations that have been identified. Neocortical neurogenesis is a process by which new nerve cells are produced in the brain's neocortex. It is important to note that there has never been a single gene mutation or copy number variation that is present in all or a majority of individuals with ASD. All of these genetic variations can be attributed as a group to the genetic anomalies which can increase the risk for ASD. Also, many of these genetic variations are *de novo* mutations. In other words, they are not inherited and must have been influenced by environmental exposures.

This article focuses on prenatal neurogenesis, but it is important to note that neurogenesis continues in the post-natal period (see Walton, 2012). Disruption from environmental exposures after birth can affect neurogenesis and synaptogenesis in the brain. As shown by Sandin et al. in the author's second reference in this article, environmental exposures account for approximately half of the risk for ASD. These exposures could include vaccinations and medications which expose the child in utero or in early childhood. Some of these environmental exposures have been linked to ASD in numerous studies. Focusing only on genetics and ignoring environmental exposures will not tell the whole story in the pathogenesis of ASD.

As concluded in this article, neurogenesis needs to be studied and understood more completely. The article further concludes, animal models studied so far do not accurately reflect the human condition. Human neurogenesis involves different cells in the brain from those identified in current animal models. Human neurogenesis continues in the postnatal period through adulthood and would continue to be affected by environmental exposures. These exposures do not necessarily have to have a detrimental effect and may offer hope for ASD treatment by stimulating neuron production. ASD should be studied in relation to both genetics and environmental exposures that affect ASD development and also offer hope for its treatment.

Review of Gerber and Offit: Vaccines and Autism: A Tale of Shifting Hypotheses

This review of published studies suffers from many problems. Beginning with their title, the authors seem to have an unscientific attitude regarding the vaccine/autism link. In their prologue, they make an opinion statement (without any references from the literature) that the increase in the rate of autism diagnoses is likely due to broadened diagnostic criteria and increased awareness. This unproven assertion should not be used as an opening statement and suggests that they have a biased point of view. This statement best belongs in the conclusion section with appropriate scientific references. In fact, recent studies have questioned the validity of this statement and have demonstrated real increases in the rate of autism diagnosed in children.

The authors fail to include evidence from my study published in 2008 in the journal *Autism*. The MMR vaccination along with acetaminophen use does indeed increase the risk for autism in this case-control study. In my study, I was able to show significant increase in risk for autism with the use of acetaminophen at the time of vaccination. This risk was not seen with the use of ibuprofen. Since this first article, I have written additional publications exploring the increased risk for autism from acetaminophen use after the MMR vaccination.

None of the studies examined for this review include the collection of data regarding medication use of the children at the time of vaccination. This is an egregious omission. Collection of this data must be done to determine if there is an interaction between vaccination and medication use that increases the risk for autism.

It is not enough for the authors to pronounce that vaccines are safe. To ensure vaccine safety, a cohort of children must be enrolled to conduct long-term follow-up studies. These studies must include the collection of data regarding vaccinations, medication use, and potentially confounding variables. To date, no such studies have been conducted for any childhood vaccinations.

Review of Offit: Vaccines and autism in primate model

This article is a commentary that adds nothing to the knowledge base regarding the cause or causes of autism. Although commentaries in general do not need to conform as rigorously to the norms of scientific articles, this particular commentary goes beyond the pale to insult parents who are rightly concerned about what may be injected into their children. Ridiculing parents by comparing them to people in the past who thought that polio might be caused by "rats, cats, fleas, chickens, shark vapors, doctors' beards, organ grinders' monkeys, and poisonous gases from Europe" does nothing to allay their fears.

Apparently, the author believes that parents should not have the right to choose whether or not to vaccinate their children, or, indeed to space vaccinations over a longer time if they feel their child needs more time to recuperate between each vaccine.

This article does report some interesting findings (Ault, 2015) regarding percentages from practitioners who were surveyed regarding their experience with parents concerned about vaccines. Practitioners report that 61% of parents who wish to modify their child's vaccination schedule do so because of fear of autism. The concerns of parents should not be lightly dismissed.

Although the author considers this issue settled with the publication of the study of rhesus macaques by Gadad et al., there is still much room for additional research. This is especially true when the safety of our children is concerned. To date, no long-term follow-up studies of vaccinated and unvaccinated children have been conducted. Only this type of prospective cohort study will provide the evidence required for determining vaccine safety.

Review of Gadad et al.: Administration of thimerosal-containing vaccines to infant rhesus macaques does not result in autism-like behavior or neuropathology

This is an important study and I was very interested in their results. However, there is a problem with their interpretation of results in the discussion section. The authors say that the vaccines administered did not significantly impact behavior of the macaques between the cases and controls. It is strange that they say that when earlier in the study they report: The Nonsocial Explore behavior was the most frequent of the nine behaviors measured and presented the only instance of a significant effect involving group: there was a significant time × group interaction [$F(5, 393) = 4.17$, $P = 0.004$]. Follow-up contrasts indicated that the Control animals exhibited significantly more Nonsocial Explore behavior at the beginning of social living compared with the 1990s Primate [$t(393) = 3.61$, $P < 0.001$], the 1990s Pediatric [$t(393) = -7.46$, $P < . 001$], the MMR [$t(393)= -2.72$, $P = 0.011$], and the TCV [$t(393) = -2.48$, $P = 0.017$] groups (Fig. 1).

In other words, they measured significantly more Nonsocial Explore behavior in control animals than in animals in any of the four tested vaccination schedules. Nonsocial Explore behavior is defined as visual and/or tactual inspection of self, or objects, with or without locomotion, and Social Explore behavior is defined as visual and/or tactual inspection of other animals, with or without locomotion (from Table S1). Nonsocial Explore behavior was the most frequent behavior seen in the monkeys and there was significantly less of this behavior in the treated animals. To put it another way, animals treated with vaccines containing thimerosal were less likely to explore their environment. I think that finding is remarkable and should not be ignored.

Due to the large number of different groups, only a small number of animals were in each of the treatment groups. There were 16 animals in the control group, 12 animals in each of four treatment groups, and 15 animals in one treatment group. The rates of autism in the US are high but do not exceed 2%. If only 2% of the monkeys in one of the treatment groups displayed autism-like behaviors or had abnormal brains, the treatment group numbers were not large enough to have seen an effect. Having larger numbers might have changed the results.

The authors did not find differences between case and control macaques in the brain regions studied. It is unfortunate that the authors did not include examination of the brain neocortex in their study. Doing so would have made an interesting comparison to Stoner et al. who found patches of disorganization in the neocortex of children with autism. Perhaps they still have frozen tissues that could be tested to see if patches of disorganization are also present in the neocortex of their macaques.

Eighteen months of age is not old enough to see all of the developmental changes that could have occurred in these macaques. Autism is generally diagnosed up to six years of age in children. Although monkeys develop faster than children do, autism-like behaviors could have developed in these monkeys after the age of 18 months.

Also, the authors mention a significant association between low-level thimerosal exposure from vaccinations and the development of tics in boys from the study by Barile et al., but no attempt was made to test for this or other similar associations in macaques.

Although this is an interesting study, it does not show that vaccines are safe for children. Monkey brains and monkey behavior are different from those of children and may not be directly comparable, and there are other problems with this study as I have discussed above. The best way to determine the safety of recommended childhood vaccinations is to enroll a prospective cohort of children and follow them over time to see if vaccinations and other environmental exposures increase the risk for autism.

Vaccinations need to be tested for several years in a rigorous study of vaccinated and unvaccinated children to make the determination of safety. No amount of blustering or posturing by government or researchers can take the place of true long-term epidemiologic research. Even if you could get assurances from the entire staff of the Centers for Disease Control and Prevention, it would not relieve us from the responsibility to conduct this research. As I quoted Abraham Lincoln at the beginning of this chapter, "You can't fool all the people all the time."

CHAPTER 8.   CONTROLLING DISEASE BY VACCINATION

CENTERS FOR DISEASE CONTROL AND PREVENTION

I know that the great volcano at Washington, aroused and directed by the evil spirit that reigns there, is belching forth the lava of political corruption in a current broad and deep, which is sweeping with frightful velocity over the whole length and breadth of the land, bidding fair to leave unscathed no green spot or living thing; while on its bosom are riding, like demons on the wave of hell, the imps of that evil spirit, and fiendishly taunting all those who dare to resist its destroying course with the hopelessness of their efforts; and, knowing this, I cannot deny that all may be swept away. Broken by it, I, too, may be; bow to it, I never will.

~Abraham Lincoln

It really infuriates me that some people continue to claim that autism is a genetic problem. I'm looking at you CDC! I suppose I should explain the difference between a genetic and genomic problem. Genetics are what you get by inheritance from your father and mother—the genes that are in your chromosomes. Genomics is another matter—it is your inherited genes along with any changes (mutations) that you have acquired. When looking at autism, certain genes inherited from parents will increase the chances of having autism—just like I probably passed on genes that increased my son's chances of developing autism. I have to live with that.

However, when one looks at the genomes of individuals with autism, they have many mutations that were not inherited (also called *de novo* mutations), such as DNA duplications, insertions, deletions, and single nucleotide polymorphisms (SNPs)—changes in a single base-pair in the DNA. These genomic changes were not inherited and most were the result of environmental exposures.

When Kanner first described autism in 1943, he could only find 11 cases. It seemed to be a very uncommon disease that no one had ever seen before. But it was about to get much more common. In the 1980s, about one out of every 2,000 children had autism. Then on February 8, 2007, the Centers for Disease Control and Prevention (CDC) in their publication Morbidity and Mortality Weekly Report (MMWR), reported that the rate of autism had increased to 1 in 150 children. In 2009, the CDC reported the number was 1 in 110 children. The autism rate is now one in every 59 children aged eight in the United States as of the CDC report from Washington today, April 26, 2018—34 times higher than it was in the 80s! It is even higher when children diagnosed after the age of eight are included. The latest data from the National Health Interview Survey performed by NIH indicate the rate is one in every 40 children—50 times higher than in the 80s—or 2 ½% of children under 18! It keeps increasing to astronomical levels and still the CDC says that it can't tell if there's a true increase, and the increased rate is probably due to better diagnosing. They won't say that there is a real increase because that would mean that we are in the middle of an epidemic—and an epidemic cannot happen in a disorder that they claim is mostly a genetic problem. How can we have huge increases in autism in just a few generations if it's a genetic disease? It is an impossibility and the CDC knows that, so they continue to promote the fallacy that autism is really not increasing that much—it's just better diagnosing of a problem that has always existed. In reality, something is causing this to happen to our children, and it's something they are being exposed to in the environment causing *de novo* mutations.

The CDC is responsible for increasing the number of vaccinations recommended for children. They are also responsible for the safety of the vaccines used in these vaccinations. It seems to me they have been over-zealous in the first regard and much less so in the second. They seem to be quite interested in the effectiveness of vaccinations in preventing infectious disease but much less so in whether there are long-term adverse effects. In this regard, there have been no long-term studies to determine whether any of the vaccinations can cause autism or other diseases which take a long time to become evident.

According to the Food and Drug Administration, "The Vaccine Adverse Event Reporting System (VAERS) is a national vaccine safety surveillance program co-sponsored by the Food and Drug Administration (FDA) and the Centers for Disease Control and Prevention (CDC). The purpose of VAERS is to detect possible signals of adverse events associated with vaccines." This is certainly a worthwhile endeavor, but how many adverse events would be reported if they are only detected long after the vaccination? Most likely very few adverse events would be recognized as associated with a vaccination unless it happened soon after the event. In fact, doctors are only told to report adverse events that happen within 30 days of the vaccination. Autism takes a long time to be diagnosed, and milder cases may not be diagnosed for many years.

VAERS is totally inadequate to ensure the safety of vaccines. It is a totally voluntary system and most adverse events do not get reported. Autism, attention deficit disorder, and asthma—three common childhood ailments that have greatly increased in frequency—aren't likely to be reported here. Long-term studies of vaccinated and unvaccinated children need to be conducted to prove the safety of all of the recommended vaccines. To my knowledge, none of the vaccines have been safety tested over a long period of time. I am especially concerned with live attenuated virus vaccines, since they produce long-term and sometimes life-long infections with the attenuated viruses. These live viral vaccines are decreasing the health of all who receive them by continuing an immune system reaction indefinitely.

Some might say that it is unethical to have a cohort of unvaccinated children to be followed as a comparison group. But there is a solution to this. Some religious groups do not vaccinate their children, and these children could serve as the needed control group. To follow a large cohort of vaccinated and unvaccinated children over a long period of time will be an expensive proposition, and there will be powerful resistance from drug companies, some physician groups, and the CDC. But we must do this—the future of our children is at stake.

In 2016, I applied for the position of head of the developmental disabilities branch of the CDC. I remember getting the call that they wanted to bring me to Atlanta for an interview. At the time, I was with my wife and her family on a once-in-a-lifetime Mediterranean cruise—I had never been to Europe before and the historical ports of call were fantastic! I was due to stop in Atlanta on my way back from Europe and asked if I could be interviewed then. But no, they wanted me to come in later, so a week after our return to the US, I was on a plane for Atlanta. I thought the interview went well and I was optimistic on my return flight to San Antonio. Weeks went by with no word from them. Finally after two months, I gave them a call. I was passed around to several people who did not give me an answer. Then I received an email that they had selected someone else. Wow, after spending all that time with them, they couldn't even let me know. Then came the realization that I never even stood a chance. They were not going to pick someone with views other than their own—they would pick someone who would tow the party line on vaccinations and not step out of place.

One of my heroes, President Lincoln, was a genius who knew what needed to be done for our country. Yet, he filled his cabinet with people who had views different from his own. He wanted to be able to hear all sides of an issue, so that he could come to the best decisions for the country, and most importantly, keep an open mind. When he wrote his Emancipation Proclamation and read it to his cabinet, they convinced him not to release it immediately, as he would have done. They told him to wait for a Union victory, which had been very few up to that time, because it would look like an act of desperation. So, President Lincoln took their advice and waited until after the bloody battle of Antietam, where the Union narrowly defeated Robert E. Lee and the Army of Northern Virginia. President Lincoln was a great man and could listen to opposing views.

Too bad the CDC does not feel that way. Perhaps it needs to be "shaken up," not in the way of our current president who shakes things up and then just spills the broken pieces on the floor. No, it may need to be shaken up and then the pieces put back together in a rational, thoughtful manner, the way Lincoln would have done.

Some may wonder about the Lincoln quote at the beginning of this section, since it is about Washington, DC. Yes, I know that the headquarters of the CDC is in Atlanta, but they are still controlled from Washington, DC. The words at the beginning of this chapter were spoken about Washington, DC by Abraham Lincoln nearly 180 years ago before he became president, and yet it's amazing how topical they still are today. In fact, it sounds like things were even worse then with the U.S. teetering on the brink of the Civil War. Maybe we should take solace in the fact that "this nation of the people, by the people, and for the people" did not "perish from the earth." We survived that and we can survive the current divisions in our country, as well as the autism epidemic.

VACCINATION SCHEDULE

It is the duty of every government to give protection to its citizens, of whatever class, color, or condition.

~Abraham Lincoln

2018 Vaccination Schedule for Healthy Children through the Age of 12 (CDC Website)

Vaccine	Birth	1 mo	2 mos	4 mos	6 mos	9 mos	12 mos	15 mos	18 mos	19-23 mos	2-3 yrs	4-6 yrs	7-10 yrs	11-12 yrs
Hepatitis B[1] (HepB)	1st dose	←—2nd dose—→			←————————3rd dose————————→									
Rotavirus[2] (RV) RV1 (2-dose series); RV5 (3-dose series)			1st dose	2nd dose	See footnote 2									
Diphtheria, tetanus, & acellular pertussis[3] (DTaP: <7 yrs)			1st dose	2nd dose	3rd dose			←----4th dose----→				5th dose		
Haemophilus influenzae type b[4] (Hib)			1st dose	2nd dose	See footnote 4		←--3rd or 4th dose--→ See footnote 4							
Pneumococcal conjugate[5] (PCV13)			1st dose	2nd dose	3rd dose		←——4th dose——→							
Inactivated poliovirus[6] (IPV: <18 yrs)			1st dose	2nd dose	←————————3rd dose————————→							4th dose		
Influenza[7] (IIV)					Annual vaccination (IIV) 1 or 2 doses									
Measles, mumps, rubella[8] (MMR)					See footnote 8	←——1st dose——→						2nd dose		
Varicella[9] (VAR)						←——1st dose——→						2nd dose		
Hepatitis A[12] (HepA)						←———2-dose series, See footnote 10———→								
Meningococcal[11] (MenACWY-D ≥9 mos; MenACWY-CRM ≥2 mos)					See footnote 11									1st dose
Tetanus, diphtheria, & acellular pertussis[13] (Tdap: ≥7 yrs)														Tdap
Human papillomavirus[14] (HPV)														See footnote 14

By my count (including a 2nd influenza vaccine injection for first time recipients and two human papillomavirus injections for boys and girls), 44 injections of vaccines are now recommended for healthy children through the age of 12 years (from the vaccination schedule presented). Additional vaccine doses are recommended (in their footnotes) for children at high risk of infection for certain diseases. Only 23 vaccinations were recommended in 1999 when my son with autism was getting his vaccinations. It seems to me that the purpose of the CDC is to continue to add more vaccinations to that schedule. They seem to believe that more is better; however, no long term testing has been done on these vaccines to ensure their safety. All vaccinations have risks associated with them—and there comes a time when the risks outweigh the benefits.

The really scary part for me of the recommended vaccines in this schedule is the number of live attenuated viruses included routinely for injection into our children. *Live attenuated viruses are designed to provide lifelong infection!* These viruses include measles, mumps, rubella, rotavirus, influenza (the seasonal flu nasal spray and the 2009 H1N1 flu nasal spray, unless they are given the killed virus by injection instead), and chicken pox. These are living, mutating viruses that have been with us for a long time during our evolution. They know how to survive, and we are helping them by providing them with mutations to allow them to continuously infect us. Nobody knows how this is affecting our health and the health of our children.

Since I was raised in Oklahoma, I am an admirer of Will Rogers. He was one of the greatest American humorists and also one of the greatest humanitarians of the last century. He was famous for saying, "I never met a man I didn't like." I think I could change this quotation a little and have it apply to the CDC. In this case, I would say, "The CDC never met a vaccination it didn't like." I like vaccinations too, but I believe that we need to have them in their proper practical relation to their public health benefit. We need to move past the paradigm of "more is better" and realize that more research on the effects of vaccinations needs to be done.

All vaccines stimulate the immune system, produce inflammation, and activate the immune system. An activated immune system can be very damaging to the brain (especially when combined with use of acetaminophen) during the vulnerable period before axons have finished growing and myelinization has protected these long nerve fibers. As I have shown in my 2008 paper, acetaminophen use around the time of the MMR vaccination greatly increases the risk for autism.

In 2016, I published a paper using data from the National Database for Autism Research of the National Institute of Mental Health. In this paper, I was able to show that using acetaminophen in children for fever of any kind increased the risk for autism. As far as I can tell, all of the vaccinations on the CDC vaccination schedule can cause fever as a side effect. From my research, giving acetaminophen at the time of any of these vaccinations would be contraindicated. This paper is available free for reading or downloading from the US National Library of Medicine at:

As the quote from Abraham Lincoln at the beginning of this section says, it is the duty of the government to protect its citizens. In this case, protecting our citizen children means providing safe vaccinations—with long-term testing—and not trying to over-protect them with too many vaccinations. Like over-protective and well-meaning parents, the CDC has wound up damaging the brains of our children.

INFLUENZA VACCINE

He who makes an assertion without knowing whether it is true or false, is guilty of falsehood; and the accidental truth of the assertion, does not justify or excuse him. ~Abraham Lincoln

According to a report published in the Morbidity and Mortality Weekly Report by the CDC, the influenza vaccine in the 2017-2018 influenza season was ineffective, providing no statistically significant protection from influenza for children 6 to 18 years old. This was no surprise given the poor vaccination effect in Australia which used the same vaccine strains and has an earlier influenza season than the U.S. Perhaps you might think that the CDC would rethink recommending a vaccine that had been proven ineffective, but you'd be wrong. The drug manufacturers had made the vaccine and they were guaranteed payment. The CDC's vaccination campaign went full speed ahead as usual.

Perhaps you might think this was an aberration, but the influenza vaccine was also almost totally ineffective in the previous influenza season as well. And yet, everyone was still told they need to get their children vaccinated in both influenza seasons in the U.S. Why? We are told that is to keep people in the habit of getting the vaccination every year. Parents are told that children need this vaccination every year beginning at six months of age, and two vaccinations for the first year these children receive it (see the vaccination schedule). Does that make sense? Children's brains are very vulnerable to inflammation in the first 12 years of life. The influenza vaccine will produce inflammation regardless of whether it is effective in preventing influenza. Inflammation is very damaging to the developing brains of children.

We are also told that the influenza vaccine has the ability to reduce symptom severity even if it does not prevent disease. However, reviewing the references the CDC uses for this assertion, I have seen that there is no proven benefit, nor even a partially proven benefit. Their assertion of a reduction in symptoms is totally based on estimates and guesswork. Then why did they still promote a useless vaccine?

When pressed, the CDC may say that it may have helped reduce some symptoms even if it can't be proven—and it's harmless. I say that giving children a vaccine that they don't need which may have untoward side effects is not harmless and is *inexcusable*. Some children given this vaccination could develop a fever or another side effect and be given acetaminophen as a treatment. What if some of these children develop autism? We don't know that it won't happen, and neither does the CDC. My research paper which shows that using acetaminophen for fever in children is associated with autism was published in 2016 in the journal *Autism Open Access* under the title "Acetaminophen Use for Fever in Children Associated with Autism Spectrum Disorder" and, as I mentioned previously, is available for free from the US National Library of Medicine at:

https://www.ncbi.nlm.nih.gov/pmc/articles/PMC5044872/

In recent years, there have been several drugs that have proven effective against flu virus infection. Perhaps we should consider more research in this area, as well as long-term clinical trials to determine what the long-term risks are from yearly vaccination to influenza. We do not know if one of these risks is autism, but any increase in inflammation in a developing brain should be avoided. As in most things, we need to weigh the risks against the benefits.

In 2017, I co-authored a paper, "Endocannabinod Signal Dysregulation in Autism Spectrum Disorders: A Correlation Link between Inflammatory State and Neuro-Immune Alterations." This paper further explained the role of the inflammation in autism and is available for free from the US National Library of Medicine at:

https://www.ncbi.nlm.nih.gov/pmc/articles/PMC5535916/

We must do everything we can to protect the brains of children before the age of 12 while their brains are still developing (see Chapter 11). Even assuming the CDC methods of securing volunteers for their influenza vaccine effectiveness studies is appropriate (and I'm not sure it is because individuals seeking medical care for acute respiratory infections are inherently different from the population as a whole), why is it they could not ask one question about autism? It would certainly set the minds of parents at ease and mine as well. I hate to prescribe nefarious intentions to the CDC, but have they thought of this and rejected it? Or worse, have they asked the question but don't want to provide the data? It would certainly prove very useful information which could then be confirmed or denied with more rigorous studies, such as clinical trials. Sadly, I believe the goal of the CDC is to promote vaccines, and I am not sure they are interested in ensuring their safety, as this might reduce vaccination rates and compromise their supreme goal.

Unless long-term clinical trials are performed on this and other vaccines, we will never know if some children given this vaccine develop autism. As Abraham Lincoln says in the statement chosen for this chapter, not knowing and asserting a benefit makes someone guilty of falsehood, even if what they say accidentally turns out to be true.

Chapter 9. Treatments

CANNABINOIDS

The legitimate object of government, is to do for a community of people, whatever they need to have done, but cannot do, at all, or cannot, so well do, for themselves - in their separate, and individual capacities. In all that the people can individually do as well for themselves, government ought not to interfere. ~Abraham Lincoln

As I've explained in my research, acetaminophen provides analgesia by activating the body's own cannabinoid system, the endocannabinoid system, similar to the way that marijuana also provides analgesia. This can be a good thing to people who need pain relief, but it's maybe not so good for children who are trying to develop their brains. A child's endocannabinoid system is an integral part of neuron development and provides a gradient for developing neurons to follow as they are growing their long axons for integration with other neurons in synapses. When this gradient is disrupted, the axons do not know where to go and end up stopping their growth prematurely and placing their synapses short of their desired location.

In 2010, I was asked by Dr. Kris Turlejski, the editor of *Acta Neurobiologica Experimentalis*, to provide an article for their special issue focusing on autism. This journal is published by the Nencki Institute of Experimental Biology. In my article, I proposed that autism can be caused by acetaminophen through activation of the endocannabinoid system. This paper "Can autism be triggered by acetaminophen activation of the endocannabinoid system?" was published in this prestigious journal and can be accessed for free through the US National Library of Medicine at:

https://www.ncbi.nlm.nih.gov/pubmed/20628445

Research I supported at the University of Texas Health Science Center San Antonio showed acetaminophen can change behavior in mice, which helped to validate my acetaminophen-autism theory. This led to publishing of the paper "Acetaminophen Differentially Enhances Social Behavior and Cortical Cannabinoid Levels in Inbred Mice." In this paper, we and our colleagues show that acetaminophen use can change behavior in mice, likely through interference in the normal functioning of the endocannabinoid system. The paper is available to read or download for free from the US National Library of Medicine at:

https://www.ncbi.nlm.nih.gov/pmc/articles/PMC3389197/

In the 2013 landmark paper "Cannabinoid Receptor Type 2, but not Type 1, is Up-Regulated in Peripheral Blood Mononuclear Cells of Children Affected by Autistic Disorders" in the Journal of Autism and Developmental Disorders it states: "Schultz hypothesized acetaminophen contributes to the risk of autism via activation of the endocannabinoid system (Schultz 2010). To my knowledge, however, no studies have specifically investigated the endocannabinoid system in the development of autism. Herein we address the issue of whether these disorders are associated with changes in the expression of CB1/2 receptors and endocannabinoid metabolism enzymes."

Later, I was asked to join colleagues in a review paper published in 2017, "Endocannabinod Signal Dysregulation in Autism Spectrum Disorders: A Correlation Link between Inflammatory State and Neuro-Immune Alterations." This paper further explained the role of the endocannabinoid system in autism. This paper is available for free to read or download on the US National Library of Medicine at:

https://www.ncbi.nlm.nih.gov/pmc/articles/PMC5535916/

What is interesting to me is that cannabinoids can be good or bad depending on the time and dose of their application. When children are exposed to environmental cannabinoids, from say secondary marijuana smoke or medicinal acetaminophen, while their brains are developing, their natural cannabinoid (endocannabinoid) system can be disrupted and their brain's neurons can be confused about how to grow. When the time for their brain's development has ended, children may then benefit from cannabinoid administration, such as the cannabinoids in cannabis, which may help their cannabinoid system get back on track.

I propose that a clinical trial of cannabidiol (CBD), the main non-psychoactive component in cannabis (which is also available from hemp), would be beneficial to individuals with autism. CBD would prop up the sagging endocannabinoid system by increasing anandamide levels while simultaneously generating new nerve cells in the brain and improving memory and cognition. We don't know yet if this is true, primarily because our government stands in the way of cannabis research. I personally hope that the government steps out of the way or even funds this research, so that we can see if people with autism can benefit from CBD or other cannabinoids.

As Abraham Lincoln states in the quote I chose for this section, the government should aid people in things that they cannot do for themselves. In this case, the government needs to fund cannabinoid research to see if it will aid individuals with autism.

I know of nothing so pleasant to the mind, as the discovery of anything which is at once new and valuable — nothing which so lightens and sweetens toil, as the hopeful pursuit of such discovery. Abraham Lincoln

I've been working with colleagues at the University of Texas Health Science Center San Antonio on two projects to show that human mesenchymal stem cells (MSCs) can help improve autistic behaviors in mice. These studies are ongoing and are showing promising results.

There have been two clinical trials in individuals with autism that have shown promising results from injected mesenchymal stem cells. I believe this is a promising treatment for continued autism research. I have been working with colleagues to find funding for a project to show that the number of autologous (self) MSCs from children with autism can be amplified in their own blood to produce an effective treatment.

MSCs have the ability to move through the blood to areas of injury in the brain and secrete anti-inflammatory substances to decrease neuron death. Amazingly, they can also transform into neurons to replace damaged neurons. Stem cells are a very promising treatment for individuals with autism.

As Abraham Lincoln says in the opening statement for this section, there is nothing so pleasant as the hopeful pursuit of discovery of something new and valuable. Stem cell therapy for individuals with autism holds that promise.

CHAPTER 10. PREVENTION:

BREASTFEEDING AND INFANT FORMULA SUPPLEMENTATION CAN REDUCE RISK

President Lincoln said to General Sickles, just after the victory of Gettysburg: "The fact is, General, in the stress and pinch of the campaign there, I went to my room, and got down on my knees and prayed God Almighty for victory at Gettysburg. I told Him that this was His country, and the war was His war, but that we really couldn't stand another Fredericksburg or Chancellorsville. And then and there I made a solemn vow with my Maker that if He would stand by you boys at Gettysburg I would stand by Him. And He did, and I will! And after this I felt that God Almighty had taken the whole thing into His hands."

One of the things I have accomplished and am I feel rightly proud is a publication on breastfeeding and infant formula supplementation. I was able to publish this paper thanks to a stranger who heard about me and thought that I might be able to help him. His name was Chris Bacher and he asked if he could call me on the phone about his survey, to which I readily agreed. As he explained to me, he had performed a large survey of parents of children with and without autism and was looking for someone to analyze the data. He was like me—a concerned parent looking for answers and had performed this survey on his own and produced an amazing dataset. He asked parents about hundreds of items regarding use of cleaning products, makeup, foods, and a cornucopia of other products.

He offered this large and unpublished dataset to me, and with it I was able to find some very, I believe, interesting results. Almost all of these products showed no association with autism in children. But two associations were most striking—amount of breastfeeding and infant formula supplementation. Breastfeeding turned out to be highly protective for having a child with autism, and the more breastfeeding of a child, the more protection from autism. I found this to be astounding! Children could be protected by more breastfeeding.

Infant formula supplementation was also very important. Just looking at the data there seemed to be no association with autism, except for the fact that more infant formula used, the less a child received breast milk. But I had an idea that there might be more to the story. I looked closer at infant formula and found they could be divided into two categories, one group supplemented by the fatty acids, docosahexaenoic acid (DHA) and arachidonic acid (ARA), and a second group where these fatty acids were not included. It turned out that the supplemented group was protected from autism, not as much as the totally breastfed group, but significantly protected. To my mind and not knowing the circumstances of any individual pregnant woman, I would say breastfeed your child if at all possible and if not possible, please use a DHA/ARA supplemented infant formula. There are many infant formulas available and you will need to read the label.

I published these results in the paper "Breastfeeding, infant formula supplementation, and Autistic Disorder: the results of a parent survey" in the International Breastfeeding Journal in 2006. This paper is available free from the US National Library of Medicine for those of you would like to read more—along with my speculation on the mechanism by which this may work to prevent autism:

https://www.ncbi.nlm.nih.gov/pmc/articles/PMC1578554/

I am very grateful to Chris for trusting me with his data and believe he has performed a great service for the prevention of autism.

Another colleague of mine, Seth Scott Bittker, published an article in 2018 titled "Acetaminophen, antibiotics, ear infection, breastfeeding, vitamin D drops, and autism: an epidemiological study" in the journal *Neuropsychiatric Disease and Treatment*. In his study, he was able to confirm my earlier work that increasing doses of acetaminophen and decreased amounts of breastfeeding in children were associated with increased risk for autism.

As a side note to breastfeeding research, it is interesting to read what Kanner found in his paper first describing autism in 1943. Most of the mothers of his 11 original series of cases were career women—which led for many years to the erroneous concept of the "refrigerator mom." This unfortunately led to the conclusion that autism was caused by a lack of maternal care for their children—a concept that has been completely disproven. But what if it was more likely that these children had been fed infant formula instead of breastfeeding? This was at a time when infant formula was not as advanced as it is today and was not supplemented with DHA and ARA. Perhaps, inadvertently, Kanner had discovered that the method of infant feeding is vital to the prevention of autism.

I hope someday I'll be able to feel that the Almighty has taken the autism epidemic into his hands as Abraham Lincoln was able to feel in the great American Civil War. I fervently pray that this may be so. But in the meantime, hard work needs to be done. The safety of vaccines needs to be proven, acetaminophen use needs to be restricted or eliminated in children, breastfeeding needs to be promoted, and if not that, all infant formula needs to be supplemented with the fatty acids DHA and ARA.

CHAPTER 11. THE BRAIN IS MORE VULNERABLE TO INFLAMMATION INJURY BEFORE AGE 12

Determine that the thing can and shall be done, and then we shall find the way. ~Abraham Lincoln

Children in some countries are kept at home, sometimes for months, after they are born. I think this is a good practice as it can save children from infections which can have adverse effects on their developing brains—especially before the neurons in their brains have finished the process of myelination. But this practice doesn't go far enough. We need to protect our children's brains for up to twelve years from infections and other sources of inflammation, such as vaccinations. Some people will say that I am an "anti-vaccinationist," but they would not be any more correct than their assertions of complete vaccine safety. I am a firm believer in vaccinations—as long as they do no harm.

Hippocrates has been hailed since the time of ancient Greece as the Father of Medicine. For many years—perhaps not so much anymore—new doctors were given and subscribed to the Hippocratic Oath. One of the most important tenets of Hippocrates to which doctors subscribed was "First, do no harm." I do not believe we are still following this tenet with the multitude of vaccinations to which children are now subjected. I purposefully use the word subjected rather than treated, because in this case because many government organizations, following the CDC's recommendations, force parents to comply with their schedule for the so-called "good of society." Parents who are not inclined to subject their children to this treatment—without question—are chastised as bad parents, uncaring members of our society, or even child abusers! If we are a free society and celebrate our freedom to the world, how have we come to that?

Vaccines must be thoroughly tested before we inject them into our children. This is not being done today. Vaccines are developed and only tested in the short-term to determine if they produce good antibody titers or good cellular immunity without too many short-term side effects. No one knows what the long-term effects of vaccines are before they are authorized, and in many cases required, for their injection into our most precious possessions, our children.

As an example of brain vulnerability in young children, a new study, "Age of First Exposure to Tackle Football and Chronic Traumatic Encephalopathy," was published in 2018 in the journal *Annals of Neurology*. This article shows that kids playing football before the age of 12 who develop chronic traumatic encephalopathy (CTE) will have symptoms much earlier than those who begin playing at a later age. In fact, the study reports that symptom onset of CTE will be more than two years earlier for each year of football played before the age of 12. The collisions in tackle football take their toll on the brain by producing inflammation. This is another sad example that shows the results of failure to protect the developing brains of children.

Our nearest relative species, the bonobo, is mature by nine years old. Even some of our recent human ancestors are mature about that time. But in our species, maturity, as evidenced by sexual maturity, occurs about the age of 12. Why does our species mature later? The answer lies in the complex nature of our brains that take a long time to wire the neurons up appropriately with long axons that require myelination. We need to protect children's brains until they mature.

I don't subscribe to the excitatory model of autism where some think that there is an excess of brain neuron excitation as opposed to neuron inhibition which then leads to autism. Instead, I think that there aren't enough long axon connections in the CNS. Since axons develop along an endocannabinoid gradient, a dysregulation of endocannabinoid signaling could have the effect of foreshortening developing axons which could prevent them from reaching and networking with more distant brain regions.

An interesting corollary of this theory could explain why more males than females have autism. Females have more axon interconnectivity in their brains than males do. Perhaps this allows them to be aware of multiple stimuli at the same time which could have made them more alert to dangers in the environment. Males on the other hand have fewer brain axon interconnections which may have helped them concentrate on one thing at a time, such as stalking prey perhaps. This reduced interconnectivity, however, would make them more susceptible to axon damage such as might occur from acetaminophen use.

Of course, this also explains why autism is so difficult to treat. Once neurons are in place with foreshortened axons, the only way to replace them is through generating new neurons through a process of neurogenesis. Neurogenesis in the brain is a very interesting subject. It was once thought that you are born with all the neurons you will ever have—but this has been found not to be true! New neurons are produced in the brain's hippocampus, and from there migrate to the regions of the brain where they are needed. Treating autism means stimulating the production of new neurons which can be done by treatment with cannabidiol or stem cells, as I covered in Chapter 9.

One of the known features of the BTBR mouse model of autism is the almost complete lack of the corpus callosum which indicates that the long axons providing communication between the cerebral hemispheres has been disrupted. If this is the true cause of autism (as I believe it is), then the BTBR mouse model could be the best choice for experimentation.

Myelination of nerves in the brain occurs when Schwann cells completely encase the axons of nerves, providing protection and increasing the speed of nerve signal transmission. This process is largely complete by the age of 12 but continues throughout the lifespan. I am especially concerned about acetaminophen and its effect on the endocannabinoid system, as well as deleterious effect of pro-inflammatory cytokines, on the brain's vulnerable nerve axons while they are still growing and unprotected. Evidence from autism shows stunting of long axon growth which I believe is the result of inflammation.

I was by colleagues to collaborate on a new paper reviewing the effects of inflammation and immune system dysregulation on autism, "Inflammation and neuro-immune dysregulations in autism spectrum disorders" which has been published in the special issue "Understanding Inflammation-induced Mental Diseases: New Opportunities for Treatment" of the journal

Pharmaceuticals and can be accessed for free through the US National Library of Medicine at:

https://www.ncbi.nlm.nih.gov/pubmed/29867038.

The Lincoln quote for this chapter explains how I feel about protecting the developing brains of children from inflammation. Now that we know that brain inflammation in children is a serious problem, we shall find a way to prevent it.

CHAPTER 12. PRO-VAXXER OR ANTI-VAXXER

I know not how to aid you, save in the assurance of one of mature age, and much severe experience, that you cannot fail, if you resolutely determine, that you will not. ~Abraham Lincoln

Some people ask me if I'm a pro-vaxxer or an anti-vaxxer. I answer them that I am neither, because that is not the right question. I am pro-children. What I mean is that I put children first and am for producing the absolutely safest vaccines that we can. I am well aware of the suffering that childhood illnesses cause. I grew up at a time when there were few vaccines. I along with most of my generation had measles, mumps, rubella, and chickenpox. I also had my share of influenza. I would not wish that suffering on any child.

Measles can be a deadly disease and should be prevented with a vaccine. However, there was an effective killed measles virus vaccine that was abandoned after the MMR was introduced. You may ask why? The answer is that the MMR produces a longer-lasting immune period to the wild-type virus. However, I have discussed in previous chapters that the measles component in the MMR also produces long-lasting infection with the vaccine measles virus. *We don't know the long-term consequences of measles vaccine virus infection.* The same is true for all of the live viruses included in childhood vaccinations.

There is a great battle raging right now. It reminds me of the American Civil War of a hundred and fifty years ago, only now it is vaxxers vs. anti-vaxxers. Both sides are highly emotional. Vaxxers claim that all vaccines are completely safe, but we know that is not true. The CDC itself is aware of vaccine side-effects. The CDC handbook on vaccinations, the "Pink Book," lists side-effects for every vaccine. However, they don't list autism as a side-effect because, because it can take years to develop and no one has done the proper studies to determine the long-term effects of any of the vaccines.

The vaxxers and anti-vaxxers are so polarized that it is impossible to even have a conversation about the issue of vaccinations. It is similar to the current political condition in this country; one cannot even start a conversation about our president and have a rational discussion of the issues. Sadly, the last time we had an issue so polarizing in this country was during Abraham Lincoln's administration and it took the Civil War to settle the issue of slavery. This is why I'm drawn to Abraham Lincoln's wisdom and hope that it will bring enlightenment to our present age.

I feel like Lincoln did in the quote I chose for the beginning of this section. I am now of mature age myself, and I hope that someone younger will pick up the gauntlet and continue to fight for the safety of vaccines. Do not be swayed by the vaxxers or the anti-vaxxers, but keep an open mind and let science be your guide. Our children are at risk, and you cannot fail.

In these turbulent times when our concept of truth is under attack and even the foundations of science are shaking, remember this: Science is truth. Our concepts of science may change over time as new information comes to light, but science itself does not change. Science embodies the laws of our universe that do not change. The Creator of the universe made the universe with science, and He does not make mistakes.

CHAPTER 13. CONCLUSION

On the day the news of General Lee's surrender at Appomattox Court House was received, so an intimate friend of President Lincoln relates, the Cabinet meeting was held an hour earlier than usual. Neither the President nor any member of the Cabinet was able, for a time, to give utterance to his feelings. At the suggestion of Mr. Lincoln all dropped on their knees, and offered, in silence and in tears, their humble and heartfelt acknowledgments to the Almighty for the triumph He had granted to the National cause.

I am reminded of a story about an old ragged man hoeing the weeds out of his potatoes. A young, sharply dressed man came up to him and said that he was only removing the tops of the weeds and that they would grow back. The man stopped, took an old handkerchief out of his pocket, and wiped his forehead. Then he turned to the young man and said, "That's as may be, sir, but they don't like it much!" Sometimes I feel like that old man. I spend a great deal of time researching and writing about problems with vaccines and acetaminophen use, hoeing out the weeds, so to speak. But authors may still keep popping up with articles on their safety and ignoring what I say, but they don't like it much!

We must do better with childhood vaccines. They must be tested for a period long enough to determine if they increase the risk for autism or other diseases that take a long time to develop. Short-term testing will not give us that answer. And the vaccine adverse events reporting system (VAERS) currently in place will not give us that answer either. I will continue to advocate for more testing of vaccines before they are given to our children.

Please do not give young children acetaminophen or expose them to acetaminophen during pregnancy. Doing so could very easily disrupt the functioning of their endocannabinoid system. Also, it almost goes without saying to not expose a child to exogenous cannabinoids, such as marijuana, *in utero* or up to the age of 12 while their brains are still maturing with the help of their own endocannabinoids. And, please consider breastfeeding your child, and if not, please use infant formula supplemented with DHA and ARA.

I fervently hope that someday we have the autism epidemic under control by these preventive measures. For those who are already afflicted, like my son, I hope that we will develop effective treatments, perhaps cannabidiol to improve endocannabinoid tone or stem cells to replace damaged neurons. On that day, I will feel like Abraham Lincoln and the members of his cabinet when Lee surrendered at Appomattox. I will drop to my knees and thank the Almighty for helping my son and the millions of others affected by autism.

Dr. Stephen Schultz, father of Matthew and Nathan, husband of Margarita

FEEDBACK

 I would like to hear from you whether or not you agree with me. You can post a short review on Amazon to let me know what you think. Your comments really make a difference, because I read all the reviews personally. I hope to take your feedback and make this book even better.

You can also leave feedback for me on my new blog site:

autismrisk.blog

Or you can email me at:

autismriskresearch@gmail.com